Keto Diet for Beginners:

TOP 51 Amazing and Simple Recipes in One Ketogenic Cookbook,

Any Recipes on Your Choice for Any Meal Time

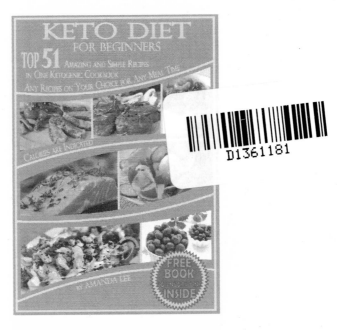

Get Your Free Bonus

I wanted to show my appreciation that you support my work so I've put together a bonus for you.

Keto Diet for Beginners:

Ketogenic Smoothie and Dessert Recipes

Just visit the link or scan QR-code to download it now:

https://wondergoodsfactory.com/landing-pages/amanda-lee-free-bonus-download/

Thanks!

Amanda Lee

Table of Contents

Table of Contents 3

Introduction 5

Chapter 1: What Is A Ketogenic Diet? 6

Chapter 2: Aspects of Keto 7

    Potential Pitfalls 7

    Useful tips 7

    Incentives 8

    Nutrients to incorporate in your diet 8

Chapter 3: Recipes. Ketogenic Breakfast 10

    1.   Keto Cereal 10

    2.   Keto Bagel 11

    3.   Eggs and Vegetables 12

    4.   Low Carb Ham & Cheese Stuffed Waffles 13

    5.   Green Low Carb Breakfast Smoothie 14

    6.   Hot Blueberry Coconut Cereal 15

    7.   Coconut Macadamia Bars 16

    8.   Mocha Chia 17

    9.   Low Carb Blueberry Muffins 18

    10.   The Quick Scramble 19

    11.   Sausage Scotch Eggs 20

    12.   Spicy Egg Frittata 21

Chapter 4: Recipes. Keto Snacks 22

    13.   Bacon Wrapped Jalapeno Poppers 22

    14.   Green Bean Fries 23

    15.   Salted Almond and Coconut Bark 24

    16.   Keto Protein Shake 25

    17.   Cucumber Boats 26

    18.   Crunchy Kale Chips 27

    19.   Bulletproof Coffee 28

    20.   Easy Guacamole 29

    21.   Coconut Butter Cups 30

    22.   Protein Shake 31

    23.   Sugar Free Peanut Butter Fudge 32

    24.   Antipasto Kebabs 33

Chapter 5: Recipes. Ketogenic Lunch...34

25.   Paleo Burrito Bowl Recipe...34

26.   Rosemary Balsamic Chicken Liver Pate.................................35

27.   Paleo Stuffed Avocado..36

28.   Low Carb Salmon and Avocado Sushi...................................37

29.   Low Carb Pizza...38

30.   Pork and Egg Pie..39

31.   Grilled Tomatoes with Apricot Jam.......................................41

32.   Brie and Apple Crepes...42

33.   Coleslaw Stuffed Keto Wraps...44

34.   Ranch Chicken and Veggies..45

35.   Rainbow Stir Fry...46

36.   Creamy Chicken Casserole..47

37.   Mushroom Omelette..48

38.   Garlic Chicken...49

39.   Smoky Tuna Pickle Boats..50

40.   Rutabaga Fritters with Avocado..51

Chapter 6: Recipes. Keto Dinner..52

41.   Coconut Chicken Fingers...52

42.   Beef and liver burger recipe..53

43.   Bacon Burgers...54

44.   Garlic Roasted Shrimp with Zucchini Pasta.........................55

45.   10 Minute Tandoori Salmon...56

46.   Spinach Chicken...57

47.   Loaded cauliflower..58

48.   Keto Cheese Shell Taco Cups...59

49.   Garlic Butter Brazilian Steak..60

50.   Creamy cauliflower chowder..61

51.   Buttered Cod...62

Conversion Table..63

Equivalents...63

Capacity...63

Weight..64

Flour kinds comparative table..64

Conclusion...65

Introduction

Do you suffer from obesity? The rising incidence of obesity is taking its toll on the health of a large population segment. While we do believe that people of all sizes are beautiful, you must pay heed to a growing waistline because being overweight is never healthy.

There are countless methods to lose weight, but traditional crash diets and starving yourself are definitely the wrong routes to pursue. This is why we want to introduce you to the ketogenic diet. It's one of the smarter dieting methods wherein you still lower your caloric intake, but do so intelligently in order to provide your body with vital nutrients and avoid complications.

A ketogenic diet is a balanced form of dieting that's-become increasingly popular due to the positive benefits it offers. It's a healthy way of shedding extra pounds because it doesn't deplete muscle, but simply works on the extra unwanted layers of fat and discards them.

In this book we're going to provide you comprehensive details regarding what this diet entails and how you can stick to it, all while enjoying your meals and shedding the extra pounds that seem to have piled on. Does it sound too good to be true? Let's get to facts and prove the benefits to you.

Chapter 1: What Is A Ketogenic Diet?

A ketogenic diet, also colloquially known as keto, is one where you decrease your daily intake of carbohydrates in order to burn body fat. This is far different from a crash diet because you don't skip meals or make them smaller.

Keto mainly involves minimizing the consumption of carbohydrates by regulating the kind of food you eat. Doing this forces your body to enter the state of ketosis. This state is where the ketogenic diet derives its name, and leads us to explain what ketosis actually is.

Ketosis – The Term Explained

Ketosis is mainly a state in which your body is forced to break fat molecules down into smaller molecules, known as ketones. These ketones are then used by the body to generate energy for carrying out different activities. Ketosis is achieved by decreasing carbohydrate intake.

The usual state your body is in is known as glycolysis.While in glycolysis, carbohydrates (carbs) are broken down into smaller and simpler substances to produce energy. As long as carbs are available, the body makes little use of stored fat molecules. However, if you reduce carb intake significantly, the body turns to stored fat as an energy source, thereby entering ketosis.

Hence, the ketogenic diet's principle element consists of pursuing a diet strictly low in carbohydrates. Apart from helping you achieve weight loss, you can also experience various other health benefits.

Keto Flu

This said, it is important to note that, like all forms of dieting, you will likely experience some form of initial discomfort.

At the outset, your body may take some time to adjust to altered eating patterns. You may experience some or all of the below symptoms.

- Headaches
- Lethargy
- Sluggishness
- Gastrointestinal issues

This phase is known as the keto flu. There is no reason to panic, because it tends to subside in a couple of weeks after your body adapts to your new eating habits. If you initiate a balanced electrolyte intake program, this problem often subsides even more quickly.

One of the key reasons people tend to opt for keto is the diminished loss of muscle common with other dieting methods. So, if you are looking for a healthy way to shed extra pounds without forcing your body into a state of extreme weakness, a ketogenic diet might be for you.

Chapter 2: Aspects of Keto

Potential Pitfalls

If you've decided to attempt keto, you should be well acquainted with certain aspects. Here are two caveats you should keep in mind.

• Do not combine keto with other dieting methods. For example: crash dieting will result in loss of muscle and nutrient deprivation, making both your body physically weak and stressing your immune system, leaving you more susceptible to illness. While this additional caloric restriction in conjunction with keto might result in rapid fat loss, the negative effects will increase commensurately, putting your health at risk.

• The initial week or two might be somewhat trying for your body. Properly attend to yourself by consuming an adequate amount of water and nutrient rich vegetables.

Useful tips

It can be too hard to adhere the diet strictly in first few weeks. The temptation to eat something sweet, tasty and forbidden is all around you and it's difficult to stand against. However, if you want to achieve the desired results, it's extremely necessary to show all your will and be strict with yourself. This is the only way to succeed in your goal. Methods of self-discipline development may become a substantial help in achieving the desired results. There are many works which are devoted to this subject, but I'd like to recommend you "Daily Self-Discipline" book by Emily Clemons. This is a really great book that will strengthen your willpower and teach you how to get rid of bad habits just in a few couple weeks and to achieve your goals.

And moreover, the techniques and tips that are presented in Emily's book are applicable not only for the diet but almost for all aspects of life. Just click this link or scan QR-code for more information about the contents of this book.

Go to the "Daily Self-Discipline" by Emily Clemons

Incentives

A ketogenic diet aids in healthy loss of weight without excessive muscle wasting. Your body will retain the capacity to carry out normal daily activities. With the addition of higher protein consumption and regular exercise, it's even possible to gain lean muscle tissue while burning fat quicker. So, if you're a fitness buff looking for ways to stay consistently healthy and fit, you should definitely delve deeper into the dynamics of keto.

Additionally, scientific research has found that people following a ketogenic diet show improvements with regard to maintaining proper blood sugar levels. Thus, patients suffering from diabetes are also potential candidates for keto. Those suffering from high blood pressure can see major reductions during diet initiation, while facilitating stability and regulation long term. Others with heart disease will find that keto tends to curb the level of triglycerides in the body while showing a decrease in the level of LDL cholesterol and even blood glucose. HDL (the 'good') cholesterol tends to increase.

Now, while this next point doesn't currently have ample conclusive evidence, research has indicated that a ketogenic diet is known to starve cancer cells, aiding in curtailing the growth of tumours. Nutrient dense cancer-fighting foods commonly part of keto only serve to bolster therapeutic claims. As you can see, the potential benefits this diet could impart are extensive.

Nutrients to incorporate in your diet

Before going into the details of recipes for preparing meals consistent with a ketogenic diet, we'll discuss some of the ingredients frequently used. Knowing this will give you a snapshot of food items best utilized or avoided.

Seafood

If you're a seafood lover, you have every reason to smile. Seafood, mainly fish and shellfish, are rich sources of protein and omega 3 fatty acids advocated in keto. But, the carbohydrate content in shellfish tends to vary somewhat. Gauge the potential carb intake by researching the particular species before purchase.

Ideally, two servings of seafood every week are recommended. Salmon, mackerel, and sardines are top choices.

Cheese

If you wondered if you read that heading correctly, rest assured you did. Cheese is actually very low in carb content and high in fat. It contains conjugated linoleum acid (CLA), a type of fat comprehensively shown to have several different anti-obesity mechanisms resulting in body fat reduction and improved overall body composition, making it one of the best foods for keto.

Eggs

Eggs are definitely on the keto chart. A large egg contains less than 1 gram of carbohydrate. Their consumption is known to trigger specific hormones that give you a feeling your appetite has been satiated, which could help you cut superfluous calorie intake. Eggs also aid in stabilizing blood sugar levels, definitely making them a good option.

Low Carb Vegetables

There are a lot of non-starchy vegetables known to be low in both calories and carbs while being extremely nutrient dense. Cruciferous vegetables like broccoli, cauliflower, kale are very good choices.

Avoid starchy vegetables such as potatoes, corn, yams, pumpkin, squash, and zucchini. We know potatoes are a staple part of many diets, but even a small serving could fulfill your carb intake for the day.

Animal Proteins

Animal proteins like meat and fish have an extremely small amount of carbs. They come in handy to sate hunger pangs and you should consume moderate amounts. Further, organ meats like liver, heart, and bone marrow are also low carb, with greater mineral content, making them good candidates. Lamb, goat, venison and even grass fed beef seem to be good options for ketogenic diet followers.

These are some of the food groups you need to stick with when implementing a ketogenic diet. They'll help you derive the greatest benefits from this form of regimen.

Chapter 3: Recipes. Ketogenic Breakfast

Here, are 51 great recipes to ensure you'll be able to enjoy food, despite dieting. We'll be sharing recipes for breakfast, snacks, lunch, and dinner so you can keep munching a bit whenever you want.

Let's start with some of the most delectable breakfast recipes that will help you kick start your day the right way.

1. Keto Cereal

This keto cereal is a healthy choice for everyone who is looking to shed extra pounds without comprising on taste.

Ingredients

- ½ cup of shredded coconut (40 g)
- 2 cups of almond milk (480g)
- 1/3 cup of crushed walnut piece (39g)
- 1/3 cup of toasted flaxseeds (55g)
- 3 to 4 tsp of butter (17g)
- Erythritol (8g)
- Salt (4g)

Instructions

- Melt the butter on medium heat.
- Add the nuts and salt to the melted butter and stir for a couple of minutes.
- Add shredded coconut and keep mixing. Make sure the bottom doesn't start to burn.
- To this mixture, add the sweetener of your choice. Ideally, it shouldn't be more than 1 tbsp.
- Now, quickly add your milk.
- Stir and turn off the heat.

Note: Do not add too many nuts as it might defeat the purpose of following a ketogenic diet.

Servings quantity: 2	Weight:	
Energy (calories):	Total = 643.00 g	
Total = 889.00 kcal	Per one serving = 321.50 g	
Per one serving = 444.50 kcal	**Total carbohydrate:**	
Calorie breakdown:	Total = 31.82 g	
Protein: 8% / 73.00 kcal	Per one serving = 15.91 g	
Fat: 78% / 691.00 kcal		
Carbohydrates: 13% / 119.00 kcal	Protein: Total = 20.51 g / p.s. = 10.26 g	
Carbohydrates mass fraction: 4.95%	Fat: Total = 81.39 g / p.s. = 40.70 g	

2. Keto Bagel

Bagels are always a satisfying choice. Far from your normal bagel, this recipe will definitely help you with a healthy and tasty start.

Ingredients

- ½ cup hemp hearts (80g)
- ¼ cup psyllium fibre (13g)
- 6 egg whites, organic (198g)
- 1 cup coconut flour (114g)
- ½ cup sesame seeds (75g)
- ½ cup pumpkin seeds (32g)
- 1 tbsp baking powder (4g)
- 1 tsp Celtic sea salt (6g)

Instructions

- Preheat the oven to 350 degrees.
- Take a large bowl and mix all the ingredients in it.
- Blend the egg whites in a blender until you get a foamy mixture.
- Pour the egg whites into the well-churned dry ingredients and mix until smooth.
- Add a cup of boiling water and keep stirring until a smooth dough forms.
- Now place parchment paper on a cookie sheet.
- Divide the dough into 6 balls of roughly equal size.
- With your finger, make a hole in each ball then press the dough onto the cookie sheet, giving it the shape of a bagel.
- Sprinkle a bit of sesame seeds on top.
- Bake them for 55 minutes at 350 degrees.

Servings quantity: 6 bagels	Weight:	
Energy (calories):	Total = 559.00 g	
Total = 1736.00 kcal	Per one serving = 93.17 g	
Per one serving = 289.33 kcal	**Total carbohydrate:**	
Calorie breakdown:	Total = 35.04 g	
Protein: 16% / 271.00 kcal	Per one serving = 5.84 g	
Fat: 74% / 1282.00 kcal		
Carbohydrates: 11% / 183.00 kcal	Protein: Total = 72.51 g / p.s. = 12.09 g	
Carbohydrates mass fraction: 6.27%	Fat: Total = 153.10 g / p.s. = 25.52 g	

3. Eggs and Vegetables

This is a fitting start! It has just the right amount of calories to provide much needed daily energy.

Ingredients

- 80g carrots
- 3 eggs (132g)
- 100g cauliflower
- 100g spinach
- 1tbsp coconut oil (14g)
- 100g broccoli
- 100g green beans
- spices (8g)

Instructions

- Add just enough coconut oil to coat the frying pan bottom.
- Heat gently.
- Add vegetables. If using a frozen mix, thaw on low heat for a few minutes,
- Increase heat to medium.
- Add 3 eggs.
- Add various spices to taste.
- Stir fry until ready to serve.

Servings quantity: 2	Weight:
Energy (calories):	Total = 634.00 g
Total = 470.00 kcal	Per one serving = 317.00 g
Per one serving = 235.00 kcal	**Total carbohydrate:**
Calorie breakdown:	Total = 31.21 g
Protein: 21% / 101.00 kcal	Per one serving = 15.61 g
Fat: 53% / 251.00 kcal	
Carbohydrates: 25% / 118.00 kcal	Protein: Total = 27.75 g / p.s. = 13.88 g
Carbohydrates mass fraction: 4.92%	Fat: Total = 28.59 g / p.s. = 14.30 g

4. Low Carb Ham & Cheese Stuffed Waffles

If you thought waffles were just dessert for breakfast, it's time to reconsider.

Ingredients

- 7 tbsp of almond milk (105g)
- 2 eggs (88g)
- ¾ cup of almond flour (71g)
- 2 ½ tbsp of coconut flour (15g)
- ½ tsp of apple cider vinegar (3g)
- 2 tsp of corn free baking powder (9g)
- ½ tsp of vanilla extract (2g)
- 4 slices of deli ham (92g)
- 1 tbsp of coconut oil (14g)
- 2 tsp of erythritol (8g)
- 4 slices of cheddar cheese (112g)

Instructions

- Preheat the waffle iron to medium high.
- In large mixing bowl, stir almond milk and apple cider vinegar together.
- Add eggs, olive oil, coconut, and vanilla extract and mix thoroughly.
- In a different mixing bowl, add coconut flour, almond flour, baking powder and 2 tsp sweetener. Whisk together.
- Now, add dry flour to the egg mixture and whisk thoroughly.
- Pour approximately ¼ of batter into the waffle iron, making sure it's uniformly spread.
- On top of the batter, place 2 slices of ham, then 2 slices of cheese.
- Add a little more batter.
- Close the iron and cook for 3 to 5 minutes.

Servings quantity: 2	Weight:
Energy (calories):	Total = 519.00 g
Total = 1368.00 kcal	Per one serving = 259.50 g
Per one serving = 684.00 kcal	**Total carbohydrate:**
Calorie breakdown:	Total = 26.61 g
Protein: 20% / 278.00 kcal	Per one serving = 13.31 g
Fat: 70% / 953.00 kcal	
Carbohydrates: 7% / 100.94 kcal	Protein: Total = 70.54 g / p.s. = 35.27 g
Carbohydrates mass fraction: 5.13%	Fat: Total = 109.57 g / p.s. = 54.79 g

5. Green Low Carb Breakfast Smoothie

For those who love smoothies, this low carb version will definitely help you stick to your keto diet plan with something delicious to sip on.

Ingredients

- 1 oz of spinach (28g)
- 50 g of celery
- 1 ½ cups of almond milk (360g)
- 50 g of avocado
- 50 g of cucumber
- 1 tbsp coconut oil (14g)
- 1 scoop of protein powder (30 g)
- 10 drops of liquid stevia (10g)
- ½ tsp of chia seeds (3g)

Instructions

- Add almond milk and spinach to blender.
- Blend briefly.
- Add the rest of the ingredients to the slightly blended mixture and blend thoroughly.
- Pour mixture in glass and sprinkle chia seeds on top.

Servings quantity: 2	Weight:
Energy (calories): Total = 410.00 kcal Per one serving = 205.00 kcal	Total = 595.00 g Per one serving = 297.50 g
Calorie breakdown: Protein: 21% / 85.00 kcal Fat: 60% / 244.00 kcal Carbohydrates: 19% / 77.50 kcal	**Total carbohydrate:** Total = 22.04 g Per one serving = 11.02 g Protein: Total = 21.91 g / p.s. = 10.96 g
Carbohydrates mass fraction: 3.70%	Fat: Total = 28.27 g / p.s. = 14.14 g

6. Hot Blueberry Coconut Cereal

Coconut is always a good choice when it comes to breakfast. It fills your appetite without piling in too many carbs.

Ingredients

For the cereal

- ¼ cup of coconut flour (25g)
- 1 cup of almond milk (240g)
- 10 drops of liquid stevia (10g)
- ¼ cup of ground flaxseed (42g)
- 1 tsp of vanilla extract (4g)
- 1 pinch of salt (1g)
- 1 pinch of cinnamon (1g)

Toppings

- 60 g of blueberries
- 1 oz of shaved coconut (28g)
- 2 tbsp of butter (28g)
- 2 tbsp of pumpkin seeds (8g)

Instructions

- Pour almond milk into a small pot and heat on low.
- Add flaxseed, coconut flour, salt, and cinnamon. Whisk the mixture gently.
- Slowly increase heat until you spot bubbles. Then, add vanilla extract and liquid stevia.
- When the mixture has thickened enough, turn off heat and add toppings.

Servings quantity: 2	Weight:
Energy (calories): Total = 870.00 kcal Per one serving = 435.00 kcal	Total = 456.00 g Per one serving = 228.00 g
Calorie breakdown: Protein: 7% / 61.00 kcal Fat: 76% / 660.00 kcal Carbohydrates: 16% / 137.00 kcal	**Total carbohydrate:** Total = 35.85 g Per one serving = 17.93 g Protein: Total = 17.41 g / p.s. = 8.71 g
Carbohydrates mass fraction: 7.86%	Fat: Total = 77.48 g / p.s. = 38.74 g

7. Coconut Macadamia Bars

If you're looking for something different, try these coconut macadamia bars. Easy to cook, they're ready in as little as 10 minutes.

Ingredients

- 60 g of macadamia nuts
- ¼ cup of coconut oil (55g)
- 20 drops of stevia (20g)
- 6 tbsp of unsweetened shredded coconut (30g)

Instructions

- Crush the macadamia nuts thoroughly in the blender.
- In a mixing bowl, add coconut oil and shredded coconut. Mix thoroughly.
- Add the macadamia nuts and stevia drops.
- Mix thoroughly then pour the batter into a 9x9 baking dish lined with parchment paper.
- Refrigerate the mixture overnight.

Note: if you want crunchier bars, store them in the freezer.

Servings quantity: -	Weight:
Energy (calories): Total = 1007.00 kcal	Total = 165.00 g
	Total carbohydrate: Total = 13.86 g
Calorie breakdown: Protein: 2% / 20.00 kcal Fat: 93% / 934.00 kcal Carbohydrates: 6% / 56.00 kcal	Protein: Total = 5.75 g
Carbohydrates mass fraction: 8.40%	Fat: Total = 110.00 g

8. Mocha Chia

Quick to make, this is for all those days when you don't feel like cooking an elaborate meal.

Ingredients

- ¾ cup of brewed coffee (159g)
- 1 tbsp almond nut butter (16g)
- ⅔ cup of coconut cream (161g)
- ¼ cup of chia seeds (36g)
- 2 tbsp of granulated butter (28g)
- 1 tsp of vanilla (4g)
- Cinnamon to taste (1g)

Instructions

1. Add all ingredients to mixing bowl and mix thoroughly.
2. Refrigerate overnight.
3. Serve.

Servings quantity: 2	Weight:
Energy (calories):	Total = 424.00 g
Total = 1024.00 kcal	Per one serving = 212.00 g
Per one serving = 512.00 kcal	**Total carbohydrate:**
Calorie breakdown:	Total = 30.22 g
Protein: 5% / 54.00 kcal	Per one serving = 15.11 g
Fat: 82% / 837.00 kcal	
Carbohydrates: 12% / 122.00 kcal	Protein: Total = 15.62 g / p.s. = 7.81 g
Carbohydrates mass fraction: 7.13%	Fat: Total = 98.79 g / p.s. = 49.40 g

9. Low Carb Blueberry Muffins

Who doesn't like muffins? Here's a quick way to make a keto friendly variety.

Ingredients

- 3 organic eggs, extra large (168g)
- 5 tbsp coconut flour (31g)
- ¼ cup of organic heavy cream (30g)
- ½ cup of frozen blueberries (78g)
- ⅓ cup of erythritol crystals (65g)
- ¼ cup of coconut milk (60g)

Instructions

- Preheat oven to 350.
- Line muffin pan with muffin liners.
- Whisk eggs, cream, and erythritol in a large bowl.
- Add coconut flour to the egg mixture and whisk until smooth.
- Wait until the batter thickens.
- Add frozen blueberries and mix again.
- Spoon the batter into each muffin cup.
- Bake 25 to 30 minutes.

Servings quantity: 6 muffins	Weight:
Energy (calories): Total = 738.00 kcal	Total = 432.00 g Per one serving = 72.00 g
Per one serving = 123.00 kcal	**Total carbohydrate:**
Calorie breakdown:	Total = 24.50 g Per one serving = 4.08 g
Protein: 15% / 108.00 kcal	
Fat: 72% / 533.00 kcal	
Carbohydrates: 13% / 98.00 kcal	Protein: Total = 25.55 g / p.s. = 4.26 g
Carbohydrates mass fraction: 5.67%	Fat: Total = 61.88 g / p.s. = 10.31 g

10.   The Quick Scramble

This is one for quick meal planners and early birds.

Ingredients

- 6 whisked eggs (264g)
- 1 cup of spinach (30g)
- 8 bella mushrooms (baby) (80g)
- 4 slices of deli ham (112g)
- ½ cup of red bell peppers (75g)
- 1 tbsp of coconut oil (14g)
- Salt and pepper (5g)

Instructions

- Thoroughly chop vegetables and ham.
- Melt ½ tbsp of butter in frying pan it.
- sauté the vegetables and ham.
- Pour the whisked eggs into another frying pan. Add ½ tbsp of butter.
- Cook on medium heat while continuously stirring.
- Season eggs with salt and pepper.
- Add the sautéed vegetables and ham to the eggs and mix.

Servings quantity: 2	Weight:
Energy (calories):	Total = 579.00 g
Total = 731.00 kcal	Per one serving = 289.50 g
Per one serving = 365.50 kcal	**Total carbohydrate:**
Calorie breakdown:	Total = 15.98 g
Protein: 32% / 236.00 kcal	Per one serving = 7.99 g
Fat: 60% / 437.00 kcal	
Carbohydrates: 8% / 60.00 kcal	Protein: Total = 56.08 g / p.s. = 28.04 g
Carbohydrates mass fraction: 2.76%	Fat: Total = 49.03 g / p.s. = 24.52 g

11.   Sausage Scotch Eggs

There are few things as good for breakfast as traditional scotch eggs; tasty, healthy and fast.

Ingredients

- 1 lb of ground pork (454g)
- 6 medium sized eggs (264g)
- 1 tbsp of homemade gingerbread spice mix (7g)
- 1 tsp of salt (6g)
- 1 tsp black pepper (3g)

Instructions

- Boil the eggs then let cool for ~10 minutes before peeling.
- Preheat oven to 350 F
- Mix gingerbread spice mix, salt, pepper and ground pork in a large bowl.
- For every egg, measure out ⅓ cup of the seasoned ground pork.
- Make patties (similar to hamburger patties) from each lump of pork.
- Place an egg in the center of each patty.
- Fold the pork patties around each egg, fully encasing them as evenly as possible.
- Place them on a baking sheet and bake for 15 to 20 minutes.

Servings quantity: 6 scotch eggs	Weight:
Energy (calories): Total = 1595.00 kcal	Total = 733.00 g Per one serving = 122.17 g
Per one serving = 265.83 kcal	**Total carbohydrate:**
Calorie breakdown: Protein: 30% / 473.00 kcal Fat: 69% / 1096.00 kcal Carbohydrates: 2% / 27.00 kcal	Total = 8.17 g Per one serving = 1.36 g Protein: Total = 110.74 g / p.s. = 18.46 g
Carbohydrates mass fraction: 1.11%	Fat: Total = 121.54 g / p.s. = 20.26 g

12.   Spicy Egg Frittata

Mmmm… you'll wanna eat a whole lotta this frittata!

Ingredients

- 5 eggs (220g)
- 4 strips of bacon (20g)
- 10–12 cherry tomatoes (190g)
- ½ chopped onion (55g)
- 1-2 minced Serrano peppers (9g)
- 1 chopped green peppers (119g)
- ¼ tsp of black pepper (1g)
- ½ tsp of turmeric (2g)
- Pinch of kosher salt (1g)

Instructions

- Mix eggs, green pepper, Serrano peppers, salt, pepper, and turmeric in a bowl.
- Cook bacon in a cast iron skillet until crisp.
- Remove bacon. Set aside to drain and cool until safe to handle, then crumble thoroughly.
- Pour out excess bacon fat, leaving just enough to coat the bottom of the skillet.
- Add onions then the egg mixture. Stir together.
- Cook for 5 to 6 minutes then add tomatoes and bacon on the top.
- Bake in oven at 350 F for 5 minutes.

Servings quantity: 3		Weight:
Energy (calories):		Total = 617.00 g
Total = 466.00 kcal		Per one serving = 205.67 g
Per one serving = 155.33 kcal		**Total carbohydrate:**
Calorie breakdown:		Total = 22.98 g
Protein: 29% / 137.00 kcal		Per one serving = 7.66 g
Fat: 52% / 244.00 kcal		
Carbohydrates: 18% / 84.00 kcal		Protein: Total = 33.45 g / p.s. = 11.15 g
Carbohydrates mass fraction: 3.72%		Fat: Total = 27.58 g / p.s. = 9.19 g

Chapter 4: Recipes. Keto Snacks

Here are some of the best keto snack recipes. Use these easy munching options between meals.

13.   Bacon Wrapped Jalapeno Poppers

Jalapeno poppers are popular worldwide for a reason and they just happen to be perfect for keto.

Ingredients

- 16 fresh jalapenos (224g)
- 16 strips of bacon (80g)
- ¼ cup of cheddar cheese (shredded) (28g)
- 4 oz of cream cheese (113g)
- 1 tsp of salt (6g)
- 1 tsp of paprika (2g)

Instructions

- Preheat oven to 350 F
- Cut the jalapenos in half, lengthwise. Remove the stems, seeds, and inner membrane.
- Mix cream cheese and cheddar cheese together in a bowl.
- Fill each jalapeno half with the cheese mix.
- Wrap each stuffed jalapeno with bacon.
- Place them on a baking dish.
- Bake for 20 to 25 minutes
- Sprinkle salt and paprika to taste.

Servings quantity: 16 jalapeno poppers		Weight:	
Energy (calories):		Total = 454.00 g	
Total = 822.00 kcal		Per one serving = 28.38 g	
Per one serving = 51.38 kcal		**Total carbohydrate:**	
Calorie breakdown:		Total = 25.85 g	
Protein: 11% / 92.00 kcal		Per one serving = 1.62 g	
Fat: 77% / 635.00 kcal			
Carbohydrates: 12% / 95.00 kcal		Protein: Total = 24.44 g / p.s. = 1.53 g	
Carbohydrates mass fraction: 5.69%		Fat: Total = 73.14 g / p.s. = 4.57 g	

14.   Green Bean Fries

If you're really health conscious and looking for a snack you won't have to fuss over, look no further.

Ingredients

- 1 large egg (50g)
- 12 oz of green beans (340g)
- ½ tsp of garlic powder (2g)
- ⅔ cup of grated parmesan (67g)
- ¼ tsp of paprika (1g)
- ¼ tsp black pepper (1g)
- ½ tsp salt (3g)

Instructions

- Preheat oven to 400 F.
- Rinse the green beans, pat dry, and snip the ends.
- In a shallow plate, mix the grated parmesan cheese and seasonings evenly.
- Whisk eggs in a large bowl.
- Dredge the green beans thoroughly in the eggs, letting excess egg drip off.
- Press the green beans onto the cheese mixture.
- Sprinkle more cheese on top.
- Place the beams on a greased baking sheet.
- Bake for 10 minutes until cheese is slightly gold in color.

Servings quantity: 2	Weight:
Energy (calories):	Total = 463.00 g
Total = 436.00 kcal	Per one serving = 231.50 g
Per one serving = 218.00 kcal	**Total carbohydrate:**
Calorie breakdown:	Total = 26.31 g
Protein: 27% / 119.00 kcal	Per one serving = 13.16 g
Fat: 51% / 221.00 kcal	
Carbohydrates: 22% / 97.00 kcal	Protein: Total = 29.55 g / p.s. = 14.78 g
Carbohydrates mass fraction: 5.68%	Fat: Total = 25.08 g / p.s. = 12.54 g

15.   Salted Almond and Coconut Bark

If you like sweet and savory, this one is worth the extra effort.

Ingredients

- ½ cup of coconut butter (109g)
- 100 g of dark chocolate
- ½ cup of almonds (72g)
- ½ tsp of almond extract (4g)
- ½ cup of unsweetened flaked coconut (39g)
- 10 drops of liquid stevia (10g)
- Sea salt to taste (4g)

Instructions

- Preheat the oven to 350F.
- Line a baking sheet with foil. Spread the coconut and almonds on it.
- Toast in the oven for 5 to 8 minutes.
- Stir occasionally to prevent burning.
- After they're thoroughly toasted, set aside to cool.
- Melt the dark chocolate in a double boiler.
- Stir in the coconut butter.
- Add almond extract and liquid stevia. Mix well and set aside.
- Line a baking sheet with parchment paper and pour the chocolate mixture on top.
- Spread evenly using the back of a spoon.
- Sprinkle the roasted almonds and coconut flakes evenly on top and gently press them in.
- Sprinkle with sea salt.
- Refrigerate for 1 hour.

Servings quantity: -	Weight:
Energy (calories): Total = 2179.00 kcal	Total = 335.00 g
	Total carbohydrate: Total = 77.56 g
Calorie breakdown: Protein: 4% / 88.00 kcal Fat: 80% / 1745.00 kcal Carbohydrates: 14% / 312.00 kcal	
Carbohydrates mass fraction: 23.15%	Protein: Total = 24.20 g / Fat: Total = 201.83 g /

16.   Keto Protein Shake

Shakes are always good for a quick snack.

Ingredients

- 1 tbsp of cocoa powder (5g)
- 1 scoop of chocolate protein powder (30g)
- 1 cup of almond milk (240g)
- 1 tbsp of peanut butter (16g)
- 2 tsp of erythritol (8g)
- 4 ice cubes (120g)
- 1 tbsp of coconut oil (14g)

Instructions

- Mix all the dry ingredients in a large bowl.
- In a blender, add the liquid ingredients and mix briefly.
- Transfer the dry mixture into the blender and mix.
- Add ice cubes and blend thoroughly.

Note: You can choose any main liquid for your shake – water, cream, coconut milk, almond milk, or milk. We recommend sticking with lower carb options.

Servings quantity: 1	Weight:	
Energy (calories):	Total = 433.00 g	
Total = 353.00 kcal	Per one serving = 433.00 g	
Per one serving = 353.00 kcal	**Total carbohydrate:**	
Calorie breakdown:	Total = 11.00 g	
Protein: 24% / 86.00 kcal	Per one serving = 11.00 g	
Fat: 65% / 228.00 kcal		
Carbohydrates: 9% / 31.00 kcal	Protein: Total = 22.57 g / p.s. = 22.57 g	
Carbohydrates mass fraction: 2.54%	Fat: Total = 26.49 g / p.s. = 26.49 g	

17.   Cucumber Boats

This is an exciting and fun recipe, with a presentation suitable for entertaining.

Ingredients

- 1 small cucumber cut in half lengthwise and seeds removed(158g)
- 4 slices of turkey bacon, cooked until crispy, then crumbled (64g)
- 1 6" whole wheat tortilla; low carb (24g)
- 3 oz of softened whipped cream cheese (57g)
- 1 slice of smoked deli turkey, finely diced (28g)
- 1 tbsp of mayonnaise (14g)
- 1 tbsp of grated parmesan cheese (5g)
- ¼ tsp of dried basil (0.3g)
- 1 tbsp of diced pimiento pepper (9g)

Instructions

- Mix cream cheese, dried basil, diced turkey, mayonnaise, parmesan, bacon and pimientos in a medium bowl.
- Using a spoon, hollow out the cucumber halves.
- Spoon the mixture into the cucumber halves.
- Cut the edges off the tortilla to make it square.
- Slice the square in half diagonally, making two triangles.
- Place each cucumber half in the center of a triangle.
- While holding a tortilla triangle wrapped around a cucumber, push a wooden skewer in one side and out the other, forming a 'boat.'
- Place on serving tray.

Servings quantity: 2		Weight:	
Energy (calories):		Total = 359.00 g	
Total = 555.00 kcal		Per one serving = 179.50 g	
Per one serving = 277.50 kcal		**Total carbohydrate:**	
Calorie breakdown:		Total = 20.04 g	
Protein: 17% / 93.00 kcal		Per one serving = 10.02 g	
Fat: 69% / 384.00 kcal			
Carbohydrates: 14% / 79.00 kcal		Protein: Total = 23.51 g / p.s. = 11.76 g	
Carbohydrates mass fraction: 5.58%		Fat: Total = 43.23 g / p.s. = 21.62 g	

18.   Crunchy Kale Chips

Kale chips have managed to gain massive popularity in the last few years. Snack on these healthy and delicious chips during movie time.

Ingredients

- 1 bunch of kale (115g)
- 2 tbsp of parmesan cheese (10g)
- 1 tsp of garlic powder (3g)
- 2 tbsp of olive oil (27g)
- salt and pepper (6g)

Instructions

- Wash kale thoroughly then dry well.
- Cut into smaller pieces as desired.
- In a large mixing bowl, add the kale, olive oil, and seasoning last.
- Gently massage and mix all the ingredients, ensuring both the sides of the kale pieces are coated.
- Space them evenly apart on a cookie sheet.
- Bake at 350 F for 8 to 12 minutes.

Servings quantity: -	Weight:
Energy (calories): Total = 354.00 kcal	Total = 161.00 g
	Total carbohydrate: Total = 14.58 g
Calorie breakdown: Protein: 8% / 30.00 kcal Fat: 77% / 273.00 kcal Carbohydrates: 15% / 52.00 kcal	Protein: Total = 9.53 g
Carbohydrates mass fraction: 9.06%	Fat: Total = 30.92 g

19.   Bulletproof Coffee

Isn't coffee something we're all addicted to? Here's a keto twist you might like.

Ingredients

- 2 tbsp of coffee grounds (10g)
- 1 tbsp of coconut oil (14g)
- 1 cup of water (235g)
- 1 tbsp of grass fed butter (14g)

Instructions

- Use your own preferred method of making a cup of coffee.
- Pour the coffee into a blender.
- Add butter and coconut oil.
- Blend thoroughly.
- Feel free to add ingredients like cinnamon, nutmeg, whipped cream, and stevia.

Servings quantity: 1	Weight:
Energy (calories):	Total = 273.00 g
Total = 221.00 kcal	Per one serving = 273.00 g
Per one serving = 221.00 kcal	**Total carbohydrate:**
Calorie breakdown:	Total = 0.33 g
Protein: 1% / 2.00 kcal	Per one serving = 0.33 g
Fat: 99% / 219.00 kcal	
Carbohydrates: 0% / 1.00 kcal	Protein: Total = 0.41 g / p.s. = 0.41 g
Carbohydrates mass fraction: 0.12%	Fat: Total = 25.17 g / p.s. = 25.17 g

20.   Easy Guacamole

A summertime staple, this one is quick and zesty.

Ingredients

- 2 avocados (402g)
- 6 grape tomatoes (102g)
- ¼ cup of diced red onion (40g)
- 1 juiced lime (44g)
- 1 garlic clove (3g)
- 1 tbsp of olive oil (14g)
- Fresh cilantro (10g)
- ¼ tsp of salt (1.5g)
- ⅛ tsp of crushed red pepper (0.2g)
- ⅛ tsp of black pepper (0.3g)

Instructions

- Peel and pit the avocados.
- Mash the avocados in a mixing bowl.
- Dice the grape tomatoes and red onions and dice them evenly.
- Add the diced tomatoes and onions to the avocados.
- Add the olive oil.
- Use a garlic press to squeeze the clove into the mixture.
- Mix well.
- Add the lime juice and cilantro and mix again.
- Finally, season with salt, pepper, and crushed red pepper.

Servings quantity: 2	Weight:
Energy (calories):	Total = 617.00 g
Total = 816.00 kcal	Per one serving = 308.50 g
Per one serving = 408.00 kcal	**Total carbohydrate:**
Calorie breakdown:	Total = 47.34 g
Protein: 4% / 32.00 kcal	Per one serving = 23.67 g
Fat: 75% / 616.00 kcal	
Carbohydrates: 21% / 168.00 kcal	Protein: Total = 10.00 g / p.s. = 5.00 g
Carbohydrates mass fraction: 7,67%	Fat: Total = 72.80 g / p.s. = 36.40 g

21.   Coconut Butter Cups

Seriously decadent sweet goodness.

Ingredients

- 2 tbsp of coconut butter (27g)
- 2 tbsp of erythritol (25g)
- 4 tbsp of cocoa powder (22g)
- 4 tsp of coconut powder (6g)
- 4 tbsp of coconut oil (54g)
- 1 pinch of salt (1g)

Instructions

1. Mix coconut oil, erythritol and cocoa powder in a bowl until smooth.
2. Add salt and stir to distribute.
3. Coat 4 cups of a silicone cupcake mold with coconut butter.
4. Pour the chocolate mixture into the cupcake molds. Make to a point to tilt and turn the mold to entirely coat each cup.
5. Freeze for 5 minutes.
6. When the bottom layer has hardened completely, pour a tsp of coconut oil in each mold.
7. Place it in the freezer for a few more minutes.
8. Take the leftover chocolate mixture and cover gelled coconut oil.
9. Freeze again for 5 minutes.
10. Pop from molds to serve.

Servings quantity: 4 coconut butter cups	Weight:
Energy (calories): Total = 800 kcal Per one coconut butter cup = 200 kcal	Total = 135 g Per one coconut butter cup = 33.75 g
Calorie breakdown: Protein: 1% / 9 kcal Fat: 95% / 759 kcal Carbohydrates: 4% / 32 kcal	**Total carbohydrate:** Total = 15.31 g Per one serving = 3.83 g
Carbohydrates mass fraction: 11.34%	**Protein:** Total = 4.32g / p.s. = 1.08g **Fat:** Total = 88.3g / p.s. = 22.08g

22.   Protein Shake

What's better than a protein shake to quell your hunger and provide long-lasting energy for the day's activities?

Ingredients

- 1 scoop of chocolate protein powder (30g)
- 3/4 cup of coconut milk (180g)
- 1 tbsp of peanut butter (16g)
- 2 tsp of erythritol (8g)
- 6 ice cubes (180g)
- 1 tbsp of cocoa powder (5g)
- 1 tbsp of coconut oil (14g)

Instructions

- Mix all the dry ingredients in a blender.
- Add all the wet ingredients and mix.
- Add ice cubes and blend until smooth.

Note: You can choose any main liquid for your shake – water, cream, coconut milk, almond milk, and cashew milk are all good options.

Servings quantity: 1	Weight:
Energy (calories):	Total = 433.00 g
Total = 756.00 kcal	Per one serving = 433.00 g
Per one serving = 756.00 kcal	**Total carbohydrate:**
Calorie breakdown:	Total = 22.36 g
Protein: 13% / 96.00 kcal	Per one serving = 22.36 g
Fat: 75% / 564.00 kcal	
Carbohydrates: 11% / 83.00 kcal	Protein: Total = 25.69 g / p.s. = 25.69 g
Carbohydrates mass fraction: 5.16%	Fat: Total = 66.90 g / p.s. = 66.90 g

23.   Sugar Free Peanut Butter Fudge

We know that merely mentioning dessert might elicit serious food cravings, but this recipe is completely sugar free and adheres to ketogenic recommendations as well.

Ingredients

- ¼ cup of unsweetened vanilla almond milk (60g)
- 1 cup of unsweetened peanut butter (258g)
- 1 cup of coconut oil (218g)

Instructions

- In a microwave safe bowl, combine peanut butter and coconut oil. Heat gently to soften.
- Put this mixture in the blender.
- Add the almond milk and blend thoroughly.
- Pour the mix into a parchment lined pan.
- Refrigerate for 2 hours.

Servings quantity: -		Weight:	
Energy (calories): Total = 3400.00 kcal		Total = 534.00 g	
		Total carbohydrate: Total = 56.39 g	
Calorie breakdown:			
Protein: 6% /	215.00 kcal		
Fat: 87% /	2955.00 kcal		
Carbohydrates: 7% /	228.25 kcal	Protein: Total = 61.82 g /	
Carbohydrates mass fraction: 10.56%		Fat: Total = 346.49 g /	

24.   Antipasto Kebabs

Based on your appetite, these can be used as snacks or lunch.

Ingredients

- spanish queen green olives
- baby heirloom tomatoes
- kalamata olives
- marinated artichoke hearts
- marinated fresh mozzarella balls
- sliced salami
- pepperoncinis

Instructions

- Take all the ingredients and thread them onto skewers in an alternating fashion.
- That's it. Serve.

    Servings quantity, calories, carbs and other values: vary.

Chapter 5: Recipes. Ketogenic Lunch

Now that we've dealt with breakfast and snacks, it's time for some healthy yet lip-smacking lunch recipes.

25.   Paleo Burrito Bowl Recipe

This is an amazingly healthy choice for lunch and takes less than 20 minutes to prep.

Ingredients

- 1 large chopped onion (110g)
- 4 chopped roma tomatoes (248g)
- 1 cup of sliced black olives (135g)
- 2 cups of leftover taco spiced beef (450g)
- 1 sliced ripe avocado (201g)
- 2 tbsp of coconut oil (27g)
- 3 cups of riced cauliflower (321g)
- 5 cups of shredded lettuce (275g)
- diced cilantro (9g)
- 1 cup of salsa (260g)

Instructions

- In a pan, sauté olives, onion, and cauliflower in the coconut oil.
- Add the taco meat along with the tomatoes. Cook until evenly hot.
- Serve along with shredded lettuce. Top with salsa, diced cilantro, and avocado.

Servings quantity: 8	Weight:
Energy (calories): Total = 1538 kcal Per one serving = 384.5 kcal	Total = 2036 g Per one serving = 254.5 g
Calorie breakdown: Protein: 30% / 455 kcal Fat: 50% / 772 kcal Carbohydrates: 20% / 311 kcal	**Total carbohydrate:** Total = 86.08 g Per one serving = 10.76 g
Carbohydrates mass fraction: 4.23%	**Protein:** Total = 121.22g / p.s. = 15.15g **Fat:** Total = 90.1g / p.s. = 11.26g

26.   Rosemary Balsamic Chicken Liver Pate

This is for those days when you want a filling lunch.

Ingredients

- 1 pound of chicken liver (454g)
- 1 cup of chopped leek; green parts (89g)
- 1 tbsp of apple cider vinegar (15g)
- 2 -3 tbsp of balsamic vinegar (40g)
- ¼ cup of coconut oil (55g)
- 1 sprig of fresh rosemary (removed from the stem) (3g)
- 1 tsp of freshly ground pepper (3g)
- ½ tsp of sea salt (3g)
- filtered water

Instructions

- Using a glass baking dish, marinate the liver in a water and apple cider vinegar solution for 12 to 24 hours.
- When you feel that it's ready, drain the liver and place it in a cast iron pan along with coconut oil, rosemary, leeks, and salt.
- Cover and cook on medium low heat for 10 minutes.
- Remove from heat and set aside for 5 minutes.
- Transfer the liver and juices to your blender.
- Add balsamic vinegar and ground pepper.
- Blend until very smooth.
- Spoon the mixture into a shallow sealable container.
- Seal container and store in the fridge for 2 to 3 days.

Servings quantity: -	Weight:
Energy (calories): Total = 1113 kcal	Total = 661 g
Calorie breakdown: Protein: 30% / 333 kcal Fat: 61% / 672 kcal Carbohydrates: 9% / 97 kcal	**Total carbohydrate:** Total = 25.33 g **Protein:** Total = 78.68 g **Fat:** Total = 76.95 g
Carbohydrates mass fraction: 3.83%	

27. Paleo Stuffed Avocado

Tasty, creamy, and chock full of healthy fats, avocados are virtually the poster food for keto.

Ingredients

- 1 large avocado (201g)
- 1 medium spring onion (15g)
- 1 tin of drained sardines (92g)
- 1 tbsp of fresh lemon juice (15g)
- 1 tbsp of mayonnaise (14g)
- ¼ tsp of salt (2g)
- ¼ tsp of turmeric powder (1g)

Instructions

- Halve and pit avocado.
- Drain the sardines and place in mixing bowl.
- Break them into smaller pieces.
- Scoop out the middle portion of the avocado halves, leaving ½ to 1 inch of flesh.
- Slice the spring onion evenly and add to the sardines.
- Add freshly grated turmeric.
- Add mayonnaise and mix it thoroughly
- Add the scooped avocado flesh and mash thoroughly.
- Squeeze the lemon juice and add.
- Add salt and mash to distribute evenly.
- Scoop the mixture into the avocado halves and serve.

Servings quantity: 2	Weight:
Energy (calories): Total = 617 kcal Per one serving = 308.5 kcal	Total = 339 g Per one serving = 169.5 g
Calorie breakdown: Protein: 18% / 112 kcal Fat: 70% / 435 kcal Carbohydrates: 11% / 71 kcal	**Total carbohydrate:** Total = 19.92 g Per one serving = 9.96 g
Carbohydrates mass fraction: 5.88%	**Protein:** Total = 27.21g / p.s. = 13.61g **Fat:** Total = 50.42g / p.s. = 25.21g

28.   Low Carb Salmon and Avocado Sushi

If you're a sushi lover, we've included this recipe just for you.

Ingredients

- 500 g of riced cauliflower
- 50 g of smoked salmon
- 1 sliced avocado (200g)
- 4 nori papers (10g)
- 2 tbsp of softened butter (28g)
- 4 tbsp whipped cream cheese (40g)
- 1 tbsp of rice vinegar (15g)

Instructions

- Heat a pan on heat and add cauliflower rice along with butter.
- sauté for 10 to 15 minutes.
- Let it rest until cool.
- Completely coat the nori paper with a layer of cream cheese.
- Stir rice vinegar into the cauliflower mixture.
- Pat the rice mixture onto the cream cheese layer.
- Place salmon and avocado slices on top, at and parallel to the edge.
- Roll like sushi and serve.

Servings quantity: 4	Weight:
Energy (calories): Total = 878 kcal Per one serving = 219.5 kcal	Total = 844 g Per one serving = 211 g
Calorie breakdown: Protein: 11% / 95 kcal Fat: 69% / 604 kcal Carbohydrates: 20% / 176 kcal	**Total carbohydrate:** Total = 49.02 g Per one serving = 12.26 g
Carbohydrates mass fraction: 5.8%	**Protein:** Total = 28.56g / p.s. = 7.14g **Fat:** Total = 70.16g / p.s. = 17.54g

29.   Low Carb Pizza

Yes, you read correctly. You can even have pizza while on a ketogenic diet. All the more reasons to stick with it, yeah?

Ingredients

- 1 medium head of cauliflower (590g)
- 1 cup of chia seeds (144g)
- 1 cup of water (237g)
- 3 tbsp of olive oil (41g)
- 1 tsp of sea salt (6g)
- ½ cup of cream cheese (120g)
- 2 cloves of peeled garlic (6g)
- ½ cup of grated parmesan cheese (50g)
- ½ cup of heavy cream (60g)

Instructions

- Remove all the cauliflower florets from the stem.
- Using a food processor, chop them into smaller pieces.
- Grind the chia seeds into flour.
- Combine the chia flour, chopped cauliflower, water, olive oil, and salt.
- Mix well until you get a smooth dough.
- Let rest for 20 minutes.
- Coat a cookie sheet with olive oil.
- Spread the dough on the cookie sheet.
- Bake at 200 F for 1 hour.
- The crust should be cooked thoroughly. If not, keep a close watch while baking it longer.
- When the crust is ready, remove from oven.
- Preheat oven to 400 F.
- Mix the cheese cream and garlic until smooth.
- Spread it on the pizza crust.
- Bake at 400 F for 10 minutes.

Note: You can add keto friendly vegetable toppings as desired.

Servings quantity: 5		Weight:	
Energy (calories): Total = 1985 kcal Per one serving = 397 kcal		Total = 1252 g Per one serving = 250.4 g	
Calorie breakdown: Protein: 11% / 99 kcal Fat: 71% / 648 kcal Carbohydrates: 18% / 159 kcal		Total carbohydrate: Total = 104.69 g Per one serving = 20.94 g	
Carbohydrates mass fraction: 8.36%		**Protein:** Total = 57.81g / p.s. = 11.56g **Fat:** Total = 162.28g / p.s. = 32.46g	

When you absolutely love bacon, this recipe is everything you'll ever need.

Ingredients

- 6 large slices of unsmoked bacon (156g)
- 1 recipe for Low Carb Pie Crust (320g)
- 1 medium red onion, finely chopped (110g)
- 4 large eggs (200g)
- 350 g of diced pork loin
- ¼ cup freshly chopped spring onion (25g)
- 2 tbsp of lard (26g)
- 2 cloves of crushed garlic (6g)
- ½ cup of full-fat cream cheese (116g)
- 1 cup of grated cheddar cheese (113g)
- ½ tsp salt (3g)
- freshly ground black pepper (6g)

Instructions

- Make the pie crust using your own recipe. Ideally, we recommend making one regular crust, but 8 mini pie crusts are fine too.
- Place baking paper on top and weigh the dough down with the help of ceramic baking beans.
- Place in the oven and bake for 12 to 15 minutes.
- Finely chop 2 slices of uncooked bacon.
- Place in a pan with garlic.
- Stirring continuously, cook for 5 to 7 minutes.
- Add the remaining bacon slices and cook 5 more minutes.
- Dice the pork loin and add it to the pan.
- Cook over medium heat until browned on all sides.
- Remove let cool.
- Preheat oven to 400 F.
- Combine meat with cream cheese, salt, and pepper.
- Crack eggs in a large mixing bowl.
- Add grated cheddar cheese and mix well.
- Add spring onion and mix again.
- Add meat and cream cheese mixture to the bowl and combine thoroughly.

- Spoon the entire mixture evenly into the pie crust.
- Place pie in oven and bake for 25 minutes.

Servings quantity: 8	Weight:
Energy (calories): Total = 3663 kcal Per one serving = 457.9 kcal	Total = 1430 g Per one serving = 178.75g
Calorie breakdown: Protein: 20% / 732 kcal Fat: 75% / 2748 kcal Carbohydrates: 5% / 183 kcal	**Total carbohydrate:** Total = 79.72 g Per one serving = 9.97g
Carbohydrates mass fraction: 5.57%	**Protein:** Total = 172.72g / p.s. = 21.59g **Fat:** Total = 306.17g / p.s. = 38.27g

31.　　Grilled Tomatoes with Apricot Jam

This can be used either as a snack or for lunch.

Ingredients

- 6 medium sized tomatoes (738g)
- 2 tsp of dried oregano (2g)
- 1 ½ oz of watercress for garnishing (43g)
- 3 tsp of sugar free apricot jam (18g)
- 3 ½ oz of grated Gouda cheese (99g)
- 1 tbsp of olive oil (14g)
- salt and pepper (12g)

Instructions

- Preheat oven to 350 F.
- Cut the tomatoes into halves and place cut side up on a lightly greased baking tray.
- Spread jam on each of the tomato slices.
- Sprinkle oregano on top.
- Grate the cheese on top
- Bake for 25 minutes or until the cheese turns golden.
- Drizzle with olive oil and top with black pepper.
- Garnish with watercress.

Servings quantity: 4 (3 tomato halves per serving)	Weight:
Energy (calories): Total = 656 kcal Per one serving = 164 kcal	Total = 925 g Per one serving = 231g
Calorie breakdown: Protein: 19% / 126 kcal Fat: 57% / 374 kcal Carbohydrates: 24% / 155 kcal	**Total carbohydrate:** Total = 43.24g Per one serving = 10.81g
Carbohydrates mass fraction: 4.7%	**Protein:** Total = 33.1g / p.s. = 8.28g **Fat:** Total = 42.56g / p.s. = 10.64g

32.   Brie and Apple Crepes

This dish scores points for presentation too.

Ingredients

For the crepe batter

- 4 oz of cream cheese (113g)
- ½ tsp of baking soda (2g)
- 4 large eggs (200g)
- ¼ tsp of salt (2g)

For the toppings

- 2 oz of chopped pecans (57g)
- 1 small sweet apple (150g)
- 1 tbsp of unsalted butter (14g)
- 4 oz of brie cheese (113g)
- ¼ tsp of cinnamon (1g)
- fresh mint leaves

Instructions

- Put all the batter ingredients in a blender and blend until smooth.
- Add a small amount of unsalted butter to a non-stick pan and heat on medium.
- Ladle some of the crepe butter into the pan. Swirl to spread evenly into a thin layer.
- Cook until the top seems to have dried, then flip it gently and cook the other side for few seconds.
- Repeat the last 2 steps until you have about 1 crepe left.
- On a plate, layer them one on the top of the other on a plate and start working on the toppings.
- Melt butter in a small pan.
- Toast the chopped pecans. Sprinkle cinnamon on top and mix
- Transfer pecans to a plate and let cool.
- Make apple and brie cheese slices.
- Arrange the apple slices and brie on a crepe and top with roasted pecans.
- Repeat for all the crepes.
- Garnish with mint.

Servings quantity: 2	Weight:
Energy (calories): Total = 1593 kcal Per one serving = 796.5 kcal	Total = 652 g Per one serving = 326g
Calorie breakdown: Protein: 16% / 260 kcal Fat: 75% / 1202 kcal Carbohydrates: 8% / 133 kcal	**Total carbohydrate:** Total = 35.57g Per one serving = 17.79g
Carbohydrates mass fraction: 5.45%	**Protein:** Total = 61.45g / p.s. = 30.73g **Fat:** Total = 138.02g / p.s. = 69.01g

33.   Coleslaw Stuffed Keto Wraps

This is a great recipe for anyone who loves to cook.

Ingredients

For coleslaw

- ½ cup of diced green onions (36g)
- 3 cups of thinly sliced red cabbage (267g)
- 2 tsp of apple cider vinegar (10g)
- ¾ cup of mayonnaise (180g)
- ¼ tsp of sea salt (2g)

Wraps and filling

- 16 collard leaves with stems removed (240g)
- ⅓ cup of packed alfalfa sprouts (11g)
- 1 lb of regular gourd meat (454g)

Instructions

- Mix all coleslaw ingredients in a large bowl, ensuring everything is well coated.
- When you have removed the stems, each collard leaf should have a missing strip from the base to almost midway up the leaf.
- Place the first collard leaf on a clean surface
- Orient the leaf so the base and missing stem strip are further away from you.
- Place a spoonful of coleslaw toward the top edge of the leaf. Put a spoonful of meat on top of that and top with sprouts.
- Roll the top of the leaf over the mixture then begin folding the sides in to prevent the filling from spilling out.
- Continue rolling and try to overlap the edges where the strip is missing.
- When complete, insert 1 or 2 toothpicks to prevent unraveling.
- Repeat with the leftover leaves and filling.
- Divide the wraps into 4 servings of 4 wraps each.

Servings quantity: 4	Weight:
Energy (calories):	
Total = 817 kcal	Total = 1200 g
Per one serving = 204.25 kcal	Per one serving = 300g
Calorie breakdown:	**Total carbohydrate:**
Protein: 10% / 79 kcal	Total = 55.93g
Fat: 66% / 534 kcal	Per one serving = 13.98g
Carbohydrates: 25% / 202 kcal	
Carbohydrates mass fraction: 4.66%	**Protein:** Total = 25.37g / p.s. = 6.34g
	Fat: Total = 59.45g / p.s. = 14.86g

34.   Ranch Chicken and Veggies

This is a classic recipe everyone enjoys.

Ingredients

- 2 large, thick boneless chicken breasts (580g)
- 300g assorted veggies cut into 1-inch pieces
- 3 tablespoons melted butter (43g)
- ½ tsp onion powder (1g)
- ½ tsp dried chives
- ½ tsp dried parsley
- ½ tsp garlic powder (2g)
- ½ tsp dried dill (1g)
- a pinch of black pepper (1g)
- ½ tsp sea salt (3g)

Instructions

- Preheat oven to 400 F.
- Line a large sheet pan with parchment paper.
- Place all chicken and veggies on it.
- In a small bowl, mix the dill, garlic powder, dried parsley, chives, onion powder, salt, and pepper.
- Sprinkle this mixture over the chicken and veggies.
- Melt butter in a small microwave safe bowl.
- Drizzle on top of chicken and veggies.
- Bake for 35 to 40 minutes.

Servings quantity: 4	Weight:
Energy (calories): Total = 1310 kcal Per one serving = 327.5 kcal	Total = 930 g Per one serving = 232.5g
Calorie breakdown: Protein: 10% / 79 kcal Fat: 66% / 534 kcal Carbohydrates: 25% / 202 kcal	**Total carbohydrate:** Total = 16.39g Per one serving = 4.1g
Carbohydrates mass fraction: 1.76%	**Protein:** Total = 178.16g / p.s. = 44.54g **Fat:** Total = 57.1g / p.s. = 14.28g

35.   Rainbow Stir Fry

Easily made and good eatin'!

Ingredients

- 1 cup cooked chicken (140g)
- 6 peeled carrots (366g)
- ½ small diced onion (35g)
- 2 cloves of minced garlic (6g)
- 3-4 tbsp of coconut aminos (52g)
- 1-2 cups of green beans (230g)
- ¼ cup of real butter (57g)
- sea salt (6g)
- pepper (6g)

Instructions

- In a large pan, aauté the onions in butter for 5 minutes.
- Add a bit of sea salt.
- Add garlic and cook for another minute.
- Add green beans, carrots, coconut aminos, and chicken. Cook on medium heat until the vegetables are cooked through.
- Add salt and pepper to taste.

Servings quantity: 4	Weight:
Energy (calories): Total = 952 kcal Per one serving = 238 kcal	Total = 897 g Per one serving = 224.25g
Calorie breakdown: Protein: 18% / 169 kcal Fat: 61% / 582 kcal Carbohydrates: 21% / 203 kcal	**Total carbohydrate:** Total = 54.1g Per one serving = 13.53g
Carbohydrates mass fraction: 6.03%	**Protein:** Total = 42.4g / p.s. = 10.6g **Fat:** Total = 65.85g / p.s. = 16.46g

36.   Creamy Chicken Casserole

Yet another yummy recipe for all the chicken lovers out there.

Ingredients

- 2 lbs chicken thighs (907g)
- 2 tbsp green pesto (30g)
- ⅔ lb cauliflower (304g)
- 4 oz. cherry tomatoes (113g)
- 7 oz. shredded cheese (199g)
- 3 tbsp butter (43g)
- 1¼ cups heavy whipping cream (150g)
- 1 leek (89g)
- ½ tbsp lemon juice (8g)
- salt and pepper (12g)

Instructions

- Preheat oven to 400 F.
- Mix the cream with pesto and lemon juice. Add salt and pepper to taste
- Season the chicken with salt and pepper.
- Fry them in butter until lightly golden.
- Place the chicken in a baking dish and pour the cream mixture on top.
- Chop the leek, cherry tomatoes, and cauliflower.
- Top the chicken with this mixture.
- Sprinkle cheese on top and bake for 30 minutes.

Servings quantity: 8	Weight:
Energy (calories): Total = 3907 kcal Per one serving = 488.38 kcal	Total = 2018g Per one serving = 252.25g
Calorie breakdown: Protein: 18% / 169 kcal Fat: 61% / 582 kcal Carbohydrates: 21% / 203 kcal	Total carbohydrate: Total = 45.58g Per one serving = 5.69g
Carbohydrates mass fraction: 2.26%	Protein: Total = 213.85g / p.s. = 26.73g Fat: Total = 320g / p.s. = 40g

37. Mushroom Omelette

If you have a thing for mushrooms, omelettes or better yet, both, try this recipe now!

Ingredients

- ¼ yellow onion (28g)
- 3 eggs (132g)
- 2 – 3 mushrooms (45g)
- ⅞ oz. shredded cheese (25g)
- ⅞ oz. Butter (25g)
- salt and pepper

Instructions

- Crack eggs into a mixing bowl. Add a pinch of salt and pepper.
- Whisk the eggs until smooth.
- Melt butter in a frying pan.
- Pour in the eggs.
- When the bottom has skimmed and the middle gelled, sprinkle some cheese on top.
- Add mushrooms and onions.
- Carefully ease the edges of the omelette and fold it in half.
- When the omelette has turned golden brown underneath, remove the pan from the heat source and slide the omelette onto a plate.

Servings quantity: 1	Weight:
Energy (calories): Total = 481 kcal	Total = 254g
Calorie breakdown: Protein: 22% / 104 kcal Fat: 74% / 359 kcal Carbohydrates: 4% / 19 kcal	Total carbohydrate: Total = 5.17g Protein: Total = 24.58g
Carbohydrates mass fraction: 2.04%	Fat: Total = 40.47g

38.   Garlic Chicken

Another tasty and simple quick fix recipe.

Ingredients

- 8 tbsp of finely chopped fresh parsley (30g)
- 2½ lbs chicken thighs (1134g)
- 5 – 10 of sliced garlic cloves (23g)
- 1 tbsp of lemon juice (15g)
- 2 tbsp of olive oil (27g)
- 4 tbsp of butter (57g)

Instructions

- Preheat oven to 400 F.
- Grease a baking pan with butter and place the chicken pieces on it.
- Sprinkle salt and pepper as desired.
- Sprinkle garlic and parsley over the chicken pieces.
- Drizzle lemon juice and olive oil on top.
- Bake until chicken is golden in color, and the garlic is lightly toasted.

Servings quantity: 5	Weight:
Energy (calories): Total = 3200 kcal Per one serving = 640 kcal	Total = 1286g Per one serving = 257.2g
Calorie breakdown: Protein: 25% / 808 kcal Fat: 73% / 2346 kcal Carbohydrates: 2% / 49 kcal	Total carbohydrate: Total = 13.29g Per one serving = 2.66g
Carbohydrates mass fraction: 1.03%	**Protein:** Total = 190.21g / p.s. = 38.04g **Fat:** Total = 261.82g / p.s. = 52.36g

39. Smoky Tuna Pickle Boats

Here's a recipe for when you need a packable lunch.

Ingredients

- 6 large whole dill pickles (810g)
- (1) 6 oz can of smoked tuna (170g)
- (2) 6 oz cans of albacore tuna (340g)
- ¼ tsp garlic powder (1g)
- ½ tsp onion powder (1g)
- ⅓ cup sugar free mayonnaise (79g)
- ¼ tsp ground black pepper (1g)

Instructions

- Except for the pickles, mix all the ingredients in a mid-sized bowl.
- Cut the pickles lengthwise into halves.
- Gently scoop out the seeds.
- Spoon the tuna salad mixture into the pickle halves.
- Chill before serving.

Servings quantity: 12	Weight:
Energy (calories): Total = 800 kcal Per one serving = 66.67 kcal	Total = 1402g Per one serving = 116.83g
Calorie breakdown: Protein: 53% / 426 kcal Fat: 36% / 291 kcal Carbohydrates: 11% / 87 kcal	**Total carbohydrate:** Total = 23.92g Per one serving = 1.99g
Carbohydrates mass fraction: 1.71%	**Protein:** Total = 108.29g / p.s. = 9.02g **Fat:** Total = 32.55g / p.s. = 2.71g

40.   Rutabaga Fritters with Avocado

This can be used as a lunch or dinner recipe.

Ingredients

For rutabaga fritters

- 4 eggs (176g)
- 1 lb rutabaga (454g)
- 3 tbsp coconut flour (16g)
- ½ lb halloo cheese (227g)
- 4 oz. butter (113g)
- ½ cup turmeric (75g)
- 1 tsp salt (6g)
- ¼ tsp pepper (1g)

For ranch mayonnaise

- 1 cup of mayonnaise (240g)
- 1 tbsp of ranch seasoning (9g)

For serving

- ⅓ lb of leafy greens (150g)
- 4 avocados (804g)

Instructions

- Preheat oven to 250 F.
- Rinse the rutabaga and peel.
- Grate the rutabaga and cheese into a bowl.
- In a large bowl, combine the eggs, rutabaga, cheese, coconut flour, salt, pepper and turmeric. Let it sit for 5 minutes so the flour is fully saturated.
- Heat butter over medium heat in a large frying pan.
- Make 12 patties out of the batter.
- Fry each patty for 3 to 5 minutes on one side. When done, flip to cook the other side.
- Serve with green salad, sliced avocado and the ranch flavoured mayonnaise.

Servings quantity: 6	Weight:
Energy (calories): Total = 4497 kcal Per one serving = 749.5 kcal	Total = 2207g Per one serving = 367.83g
Calorie breakdown: Protein: 11% / 491 kcal Fat: 73% / 3302 kcal Carbohydrates: 16% / 701 kcal	**Total carbohydrate:** Total = 186.37g Per one serving = 31.06g
Carbohydrates mass fraction: 8.44%	**Protein:** Total = 124.12g / p.s. = 20.69g **Fat:** Total = 379.42g / p.s. = 63.24g

Chapter 6: Recipes. Keto Dinner

And the moment we've all been waiting for… dinner!

41.   Coconut Chicken Fingers

Tasty tender tropical goodness!

Ingredients

- 1 egg (44g)
- 1 pound of boneless, skinless chicken tenders (454g)
- ⅛ tsp of cinnamon
- 1 cup unsweetened shredded coconut (80g)
- ½ cup cashew flour (69g)
- ¼ tsp garlic powder (1g)
- ¼ tsp salt (2g)
- ¼ tsp pepper (1g)

Instructions

- Preheat oven to 375 F.
- Line a baking sheet with parchment paper.
- Beat the egg in a bowl and set aside.
- In another bowl, add coconut flakes and spices, along with the cashew flour.
- Dip the chicken tenders in the egg then dredge in the flour mixture.
- Arrange the tenders on the baking sheet, spaced evenly.
- Bake for 15 to 20 minutes.

Servings quantity: 2	Weight:
Energy (calories): Total = 1248 kcal Per one serving = 624 kcal	Total = 649g Per one serving = 324.5g
Calorie breakdown: Protein: 37% / 464 kcal Fat: 51% / 638 kcal Carbohydrates: 12% / 146 kcal	**Total carbohydrate:** Total = 36.16g Per one serving = 18.08g
Carbohydrates mass fraction: 5.57 %	**Protein:** Total = 111.12g / p.s. = 55.56g **Fat:** Total = 75g / p.s. = 37.5g

42.   Beef and liver burger recipe

Count on making this a permanent part of your repertoire, because this burger is definitely that yummy.

Ingredients

- ¼ lb chicken livers (113g)
- 1 ¼ lbs ground beef (567g)
- ½ medium peeled red onion (55g)
- 1 tsp poultry seasoning (2g)
- 1 ½ tsp coriander (1g)
- 1 tsp sea salt (6g)
- 1 tsp ground black pepper (3g)

Instructions

- In a food processor, add the red onion and chicken livers.
- Pulse it until you get a smooth paste.
- Add the ground beef and all the spices.
- Pulse the food processor until the texture is not quite smooth.
- Shape this mixture into four patties, 4" in diameter.
- Grill to your liking!

Servings quantity: 4	Weight:
Energy (calories): Total = 1612 kcal Per one serving = 403 kcal	Total = 747g Per one serving = 186.75g
Calorie breakdown: Protein: 31% / 501 kcal Fat: 67% / 1075 kcal Carbohydrates: 2% / 34 kcal	**Total carbohydrate:** Total = 9.27g Per one serving = 2.32g
Carbohydrates mass fraction: 1.24 %	**Protein:** Total = 117.79g / p.s. = 29.45g **Fat:** Total = 119.18g / p.s. = 29.80g

43.   Bacon Burgers

Simple yet heavenly marriage of beef and bacon. Need we say more?

Ingredients

- 2 eggs (88g)
- 4 slices of uncooked bacon (104g)
- 2 lb of ground beef (907g)
- ½ tsp of chipotle chili powder (1g)
- Salt (9g)

Instructions

- Chop the bacon into a variety of sizes, from medium to minced.
- Add the bacon to a large bowl, along with the chili pepper and a touch of salt.
- Mix thoroughly.
- Add the ground beef.
- Mix thoroughly while salting to taste.
- Form into patties.
- Heat the grill to 450 F.
- Grill the patties over direct heat for 2 per side.
- Move them to indirect heat and grill for another 3 to 4 minutes per side.

Servings quantity: 6	Weight:
Energy (calories): Total = 2857 kcal Per one serving = 476.17 kcal	Total = 1110g Per one serving = 185g
Calorie breakdown: Protein: 27% / 776 kcal Fat: 73% / 2081 kcal Carbohydrates: 0.2% / 7 kcal	**Total carbohydrate:** Total = 2.19g Per one serving =0.37g
Carbohydrates mass fraction: 0.2 %	**Protein:** Total = 180.04g / p.s. = 30g **Fat:** Total = 230.85g / p.s. = 38.46g

44.   Garlic Roasted Shrimp with Zucchini Pasta

Pasta and keto aren't common bedfellows, but variety is the spice of life. So enjoy this one no more than once a week.

Ingredients

- 8 oz peeled shrimp (227g)
- 2 medium sized boxes of zucchini rotini (640g)
- 1 lemon zest (58g)
- 2 tbsp of melted butter (28g)
- 2 cloves of minced garlic (6g)
- 2 tbsp olive oil (27g)
- ¼ tsp salt (2g)
- fresh ground pepper to taste (2g)

Instructions

- Preheat oven to 400 F.
- In a baking dish, mix all the ingredients except for the pasta.
- Bake for 8 to 10 minutes, stirring the mixture thoroughly about halfway.
- In a large pot, bring water to a boil and add the pasta.
- Cook until al dente and drain well.
- Ensure the shrimp has been cooked thoroughly.
- When complete, add the pasta. Toss it and serve.

Servings quantity: 4	Weight:
Energy (calories): Total = 1347 kcal Per one serving = 336.75 kcal	Total = 1030g Per one serving = 257.5g
Calorie breakdown: Protein: 24% / 327 kcal Fat: 48% / 647 kcal Carbohydrates: 28% / 371 kcal	**Total carbohydrate:** Total = 93.95g Per one serving = 23.48g
Carbohydrates mass fraction: 2.27 %	**Protein:** Total = 85.71g / p.s. = 21.43g **Fat:** Total = 73.37g / p.s. = 18.34g

45.   10 Minute Tandoori Salmon

When you're in a rush but need something flavor-packed for dinner, this will be your go-to recipe.

Ingredients

- 1 pound salmon (454g)
- 2 tsp of paprika (5g)
- 3 tsp mustard oil (14g)
- 1 tsp of coriander powder (1g)
- ¼ tsp ginger powder (1g)
- 1 tsp of garlic powder (3g)
- 1 tsp of chilli powder (3g)
- ½ tsp turmeric (2g)
- ½ tsp salt (3g)
- ½ tsp black pepper (2g)

Instructions

- Preheat oven to 425 F.
- Line a baking sheet with foil.
- Combine all spices in a bowl and mix well.
- Pour in the mustard oil. Beat to create a paste.
- Rub this paste on the salmon.
- Place the salmon on the baking sheet.
- Bake 4 to 6 minutes for every ½ inch of thickness.

Servings quantity: 2	Weight:
Energy (calories): Total = 738 kcal Per one serving = 369 kcal	Total = 485g Per one serving = 242.5g
Calorie breakdown: Protein: 54.5% / 403 kcal Fat: 42% / 309 kcal Carbohydrates: 3.5% / 27 kcal	**Total carbohydrate:** Total = 8.72g Per one serving = 4.36g
Carbohydrates mass fraction: 1.8%	**Protein:** Total = 95g / p.s. = 47.5g **Fat:** Total = 34.61g / p.s. = 17.30g

46.   Spinach Chicken

Looking for an easy dinner recipe when you're not in the mood to spend too much time in the kitchen? Try this.

Ingredients

- 2 ½ lb chicken cut into bite sized pieces (1134g)
- ½ bag of frozen spinach (142g)
- ½ pack of sliced mushrooms (113g)
- 1 medium onion (110g)
- basil (1g)
- butter (28g)
- garlic powder (10g)
- 1 lemon (58g)
- salt & pepper (23g)

Instructions

- Add butter to a large skillet.
- Add the chopped onion and mushrooms. sauté until onions are translucent.
- Mix well, then add the chopped chicken. Cook thoroughly.
- Add salt, pepper, basil and garlic powder to taste.
- Finally, add spinach and cook until wilted.
- Squeeze lemon juice on top and serve.

Servings quantity: 6	Weight:
Energy (calories): Total = 1581 kcal Per one serving = 263.5 kcal	Total = 1644g Per one serving = 274g
Calorie breakdown: Protein: 65% / 1022 kcal Fat: 27% / 430 kcal Carbohydrates: 8% / 131 kcal	**Total carbohydrate:** Total = 38.1g Per one serving = 6.35g
Carbohydrates mass fraction: 2.32%	**Protein:** Total = 244.5g / p.s. = 40.75g **Fat:** Total = 47.85g / p.s. = 7.98g

47.   Loaded cauliflower

One of the best low carb comfort foods ever!

Ingredients

- 2 slices of fried and crumbled bacon (23g)
- 1 lb cauliflower florets (454g)
- 4 oz of sour cream (113g)
- 2 tbsp of snipped chives (6g)
- 3 tbsp butter (43g)
- 1 cup grated cheddar cheese (113g)
- ¼ tsp garlic powder (1g)
- salt and pepper to taste (4g)

Instructions

- Cut the cauliflower into florets and put them in a bowl.
- Add 2 tbsp of water and microwave for 5 to 8 minutes.
- Drain the excess water and let sit uncovered until cool.
- Blend in a food processor until it gets fluffy.
- Add garlic powder, butter, sour cream. Blend until smooth.
- Place the mashed cauliflower in a fresh bowl, then add most of the chives.
- Add half of the cheddar cheese and season with salt and pepper.
- Top the loaded cauliflower with the remaining cheese, chives and bacon.
- Microwave for 2 to 3 minutes.

Servings quantity: 3	Weight:
Energy (calories): Total = 1145 kcal Per one serving = 381.67 kcal	Total = 756g Per one serving = 252g
Calorie breakdown: Protein: 16% / 182 kcal Fat: 73% / 840 kcal Carbohydrates: 11% / 125 kcal	**Total carbohydrate:** Total = 38.1g Per one serving = 6.35g
Carbohydrates mass fraction: 5.04%	**Protein:** Total = 48.4g / p.s. = 16.13g **Fat:** Total = 94.2g / p.s. = 31.4g

48. Keto Cheese Shell Taco Cups

Isn't the name cheesy enough to give this recipe a try?

Ingredients

For cheese cups

- 8 slices of your preferred cheese (239g)

For salsa

- 2 diced roma tomatoes (124g)
- 3 tbsp of diced red onion (30g)
- ½ finely diced fresh jalapeno (7g)
- 3 tbsp cilantro (3g)
- 1 tbsp lime juice (15g)

Instructions

- Preheat oven to 375 F.
- Line a baking sheet with parchment paper and place the cheese slices on it.
- Bake for 5 minutes.
- Remove the baking sheet and let cool slightly.
- Carefully remove the slices and place them in a muffin tin so they take on the cup's shape.
- Let them fully cool.

Making the salsa

- In a fresh bowl, add onions, roma tomatoes, cilantro, jalapenos and lime juice.
- Mix well.
- Place in the fridge for 30 minutes.
- Fill the cups with salsa filling and enjoy.

Servings quantity: 2 (4 cheese cups per serving)	Weight:
Energy (calories): Total = 876 kcal Per one serving = 438 kcal	Total = 403g Per one serving = 201.5g
Calorie breakdown: Protein: 27% / 238 kcal Fat: 68% / 599 kcal Carbohydrates: 4% / 39 kcal	**Total carbohydrate:** Total = 10.98g Per one serving = 5.49g
Carbohydrates mass fraction: 2.72%	**Protein:** Total = 56.45g / p.s. = 28.22g **Fat:** Total = 68.16g / p.s. = 34.08g

49.   Garlic Butter Brazilian Steak

Just 20 minutes to glory.

Ingredients

- 1 ½ lbs of steak, trimmed and cut evenly into 4 pieces (680g)
- 1 tbsp chopped fresh flat-leaf parsley (4g)
- 2 tbsp canola oil or vegetable oil (27g)
- 6 medium cloves of garlic (18g)
- 4 tbsp unsalted butter (56g)
- kosher salt (3g)
- freshly ground black pepper (1g)

Instructions

- Peel the garlic cloves then smash them using the side of your knife.
- Sprinkle the garlic with salt and mince it.
- Pat the steak dry, then season it slightly on both the sides with salt and pepper.
- Heat a heavy skillet on medium.
- Add the oil and heat until it begins to simmer.
- Add the steaks and brown on both sides.
- Transfer the steaks to a plate. Cover and rest.
- In an 8" skillet, melt butter on low heat.
- Add garlic and cook, tossing frequently until evenly golden in color.
- Slice the steaks and spoon the garlic butter on top.
- Garnish with parsley and serve.

Servings quantity: 4		Weight:	
Energy (calories): Total = 1924 kcal Per one serving = 481 kcal		Total = 789g Per one serving = 197.25g	
Calorie breakdown: Protein: 40% / 768 kcal Fat: 59% / 1144 kcal Carbohydrates: 1% / 25 kcal		**Total carbohydrate:** Total = 6.58g Per one serving = 1.65g	
Carbohydrates mass fraction: 0.8%		**Protein:** Total = 192.52g / p.s. = 48.13g **Fat:** Total = 127.19g / p.s. = 31.8g	

50.   Creamy cauliflower chowder

Once in awhile, it's just nice having soup for dinner, isn't it?

Ingredients

- 1 head of cauliflower cut into small florets (588g)
- ¾ cup diced carrots (96g)
- ½ cup diced onion (80g)
- 1 cup milk (244g)
- 1 tbsp butter (14g)
- ¼ cup cream cheese (58g)
- 5 cloves of minced garlic (15g)
- ½ tsp dried oregano (1g)
- 1 tsp freshly ground pepper (2g)
- salt to taste (6g)
- olive oil (14g) and 3 strips of cooked bacon (15g) for topping

Instructions

- Heat butter in a soup pot.
- Add onion and garlic and sauté for a few minutes.
- Add cauliflower, carrots, milk, pepper, salt, and oregano.
- Bring this mixture to boil and then reduce heat to a simmer.
- After the cauliflower is tender, remove from heat and pour the mixture into a blender.
- Blend soup until creamy then pour it back in the pot.
- Add a cup of water along with cream cheese.
- Simmer for 5 to 10 minutes and then turn off heat.
- Top with olive oil and bacon.

Servings quantity: 4	Weight:
Energy (calories): Total = 863 kcal Per one serving = 215.75 kcal	Total = 1133g Per one serving = 283.25g
Calorie breakdown: Protein: 10% / 87 kcal Fat: 61% / 522 kcal Carbohydrates: 29% / 253 kcal	**Total carbohydrate:** Total = 67.65g Per one serving = 16.91g
Carbohydrates mass fraction: 5.97%	**Protein:** Total = 27.15g / p.s. = 6.79g **Fat:** Total = 59.41g / p.s. = 14.85g

51.   Buttered Cod

A simple finale.

Ingredients

- 1 ½ lbs cod (680g)
- 6 tbsp unsalted butter (84g)

For the Seasoning-

- a few lemon slices (21g)
- ¼ tsp garlic powder (1g)
- ¾ tsp paprika (2g)
- ½ tsp salt (3g)
- ¼ tsp ground pepper (1g)
- herbs, parsley or cilantro (3g)

Instructions

- Mix all the seasoning ingredients in a small bowl.
- As desired, cut the cod into smaller pieces.
- Season with the mix.
- Melt butter in a large skillet on medium heat.
- Add the cod and cook for 2 minutes.
- Turn the cod, top with the leftover butter and continue cooking for 3 to 4 minutes.
- Drizzle with fresh lemon juice and serve.

Servings quantity: 2	Weight:
Energy (calories): Total = 905 kcal Per one serving = 452.5 kcal	Total = 795g Per one serving = 397.5g
Calorie breakdown: Protein: 50% / 457 kcal Fat: 49% / 445 kcal Carbohydrates: 1% / 11 kcal	**Total carbohydrate:** Total = 4.08g Per one serving = 2.04g
Carbohydrates mass fraction: 0.5%	**Protein:** Total = 107.45g / p.s. = 53.73g **Fat:** Total = 49.41g / p.s. = 24.71g

Conversion Table

Equivalents

U.S.	U.S.
16 tablespoons	1 cup
12 tablespoons	3/4 cup
10 tablespoons + 2 teaspoons	2/3 cup
8 tablespoons	1/2 cup
6 tablespoons	3/8 cup
5 tablespoons + 1 teaspoon	1/3 cup
4 tablespoons	1/4 cup
2 tablespoons + 2 teaspoons	1/6 cup
2 tablespoons	1/8 cup
1 tablespoon	1/16 cup
1 pint	2 cups
1 quart	2 pints
1 tablespoon	3 teaspoons
1 cup	48 teaspoons
1 cup	16 tablespoons

Capacity

U.S.	METRIC
1/5 teaspoon	1 ml
1 teaspoon (tsp)	5 ml
1 tablespoon (tbsp)	15 ml
1 fluid oz.	30 ml
1/5 cup	50 ml
1/4 cup	60 ml
1/3 cup	80 ml
3.4 fluid oz.	100 ml
1/2 cup	120 ml
2/3 cup	160 ml
3/4 cup	180 ml
1 cup	240 ml
1 pint (2 cups)	480 ml
1 quart (4 cups)	.95 liter
34 fluid oz.	1 liter
4.2 cups	1 liter
2.1 pints	1 liter
1.06 quarts	1 liter
.26 gallon	1 liter
4 quarts (1 gallon)	3.8 liters

Weight

U.S.	METRIC
.035 ounce	1 gram
0.5 oz.	14 grams
1 oz.	28 grams
1/4 pound (lb)	113 grams
1/3 pound (lb)	151 grams
1/2 pound (lb)	227 grams
1 pound (lb)	454 grams
1.10 pounds (lbs)	500 grams
2.205 pounds (lbs)	1 kilogram
35 oz.	1 kilogram

Flour kinds comparative table

Serv.size: 1 cup	Calories	Carbs	Protein	Fat	Weight
Almond flour	640 kcal	20 g	24 g	56 g	100 g
Hazelnut flour	720 kcal	20 g	16 g	68 g	95 g
Coconut flour	480 kcal	64 g	16 g	16 g	115 g
Chickpea flour	440 kcal	72 g	24 g	8 g	90 g
Amaranth flour	440 kcal	80 g	16 g	8 g	108 g
Rice flour	580 kcal	128 g	8.8 g	2.4 g	150 g

Conclusion

Now that you have these recipes, are you all set to follow a ketogenic diet? With so much diversity, keto shouldn't be a hassle whatsoever.

You can mix and match these recipes and explore other options. Variety will keep your palate entertained and your cravings in check. Keep in mind the amount of calories you're consuming, especially from carbs. With a small amount of effort and some persistence, your adherence to a ketogenic diet will result in increased health, vitality, and significant weight loss in a relatively brief period of time.

We know losing weight isn't an easy task and there are plenty of dieting mistakes you have, and can, make. When you opt for keto, you'll be able to shed pounds in a systematic manner while retaining lean muscle mass and without depriving yourself of good food.

We hope you follow these recipes and see how useful (and tasty!) they are.

Dear Reader,

Thank you again for purchasing this book!
I hope this book was helpful for you.

Finally, if you enjoyed this book, I'd highly appreciate if you make a favor and leave a review for this book on Amazon.

The opinion of every reader is very important for me. It helps me to make my books better and more useful.

Also, your review will be really useful for other customers! Most of the customers consider reviews are the most important factors which can help them to choose a book.

To leave a review, you can just go to the link or scan QR-code:
https://www.amazon.com/Keto-Diet-Beginners-Ketogenic-Cookbook/dp/1522000690/#customerReviews

The process only takes a minute or so.

Thanks in advance for your time, and thanks again for choosing my book.

And, please, don't forget to receive your free bonus on the next page.

I wish you all the best.

Sincerely yours,
Amanda Lee

REMINDER:

Get Your Free Bonus

I wanted to show my appreciation that you support my work so I've put together a bonus for you.

Keto Diet for Beginners:

Ketogenic Smoothie and Dessert Recipes

Just visit the link or scan QR-code to download it now:

https://wondergoodsfactory.com/landing-pages/amanda-lee-free-bonus-download/

Thanks!

Amanda Lee

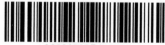

Made in the USA
Columbia, SC
01 April 2018